Slow Cooker Cookbook

Basic Recipes You Can Make in a Crockpot

Copyright © 2020

All rights reserved.

DEDICATION

The author and publisher have provided this e-book to you for your personal use only. You may not make this e-book publicly available in any way. Copyright infringement is against the law. If you believe the copy of this e-book you are reading infringes on the author's copyright, please notify the publisher at: https://us.macmillan.com/piracy

Contents

Rice & Noodles 1

    Chinese Fried Rice *2*

    Teriyaki Chicken And Rice *4*

    Vegetarian "Bone" Broth *7*

    Pork Ramen *11*

Chicken 14

    Honey Teriyaki Chicken *15*

    Orange Chicken *18*

    Cashew Chicken *20*

    Hainanese Chicken *23*

Meat 25

Slow Cooker Broccoli Beef 26

Slow Cooker Sesame Beef 31

Slow Cooker Sweet & Sour Meatballs 34

Slow Cooker Asian Pulled Pork..38

Vegetables & Tofu..40

Slow Cooked Asian Vegetables 41

Slow Cooker Asian Greens (gluten free) 43

Orange-Teriyaki Tofu 45

Tofu Lo Mein 47

Rice & Noodles

Chinese Fried Rice

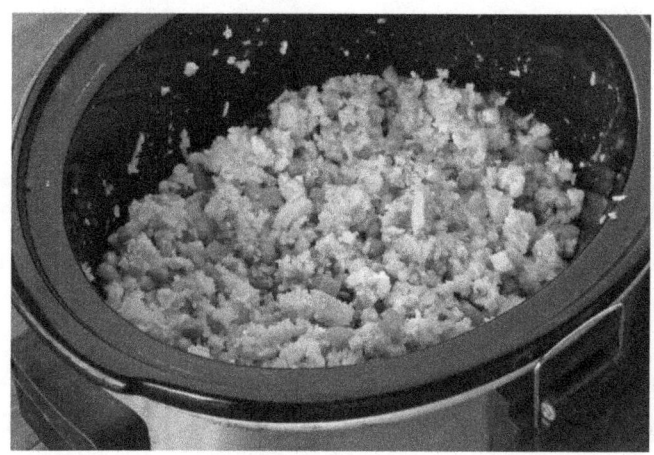

This time-saving version will have coming home to ready-made fried rice!

Prep Time: 10 mins

Cook Time: 2 hrs 45 mins

Total Time: 2 hrs 55 mins

Ingredients

1 pound cooked chicken, ham or pork , cut into 1/4 inch or so pieces (vegetarian/vegan: omit or use a firm soy substitute like tempeh)

2 cups uncooked jasmine rice , **must use medium to long-grained rice or the consistency will by mushy

12 ounce bag frozen peas, carrots and corn medley

2 cloves garlic ,minced

3 1/4 cups chicken broth (vegetarian/vegan: use vegetable broth)

2 tablespoons soy sauce

1 teaspoon salt

2 tablespoons toasted sesame oil

2 large eggs ,lightly beaten with fork (vegan: omit or use tofu)

4 green onions ,sliced

Instructions

1. Place the chicken in a single layer in the slow cooker followed by the rice, then the frozen vegetables and garlic.
2. In a bowl, stir together the chicken broth, soy sauce, salt and sesame oil. Pour it over the vegetables.
3. Cook on HIGH for 2 hours. Pour the eggs over the vegetables, close the lid and let it cook for another 45 mins. Stir the mixture, fluffing the rice with a fork. Stir in the green onions.
4. Serve with additional soy sauce and sesame oil.

Teriyaki Chicken And Rice

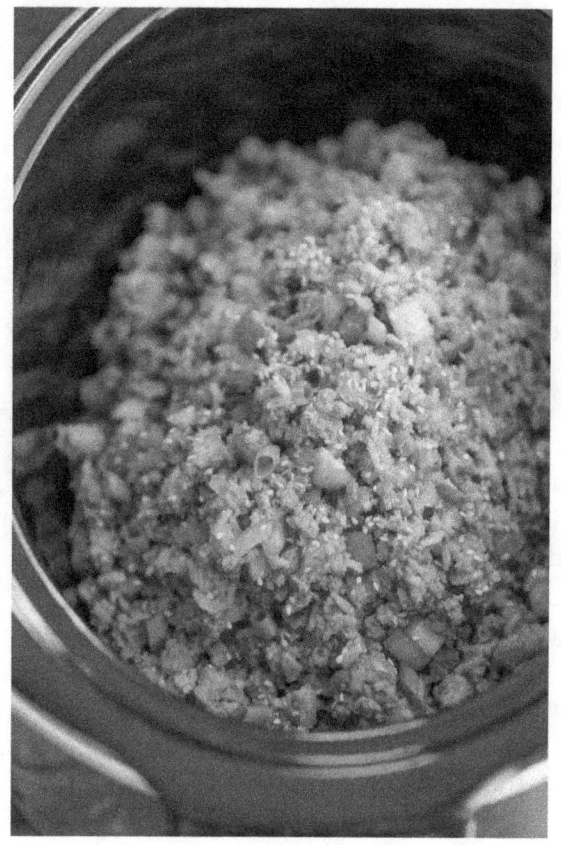

Yield: 8 servings

Prep Time: 15 mins

Cook Time: 4 hours 5 mins

Total Time: 4 HOURS 20 MINS

Saucy chicken, rice and veggies come together so easily right in the crockpot. Sure to be a weeknight staple!

Ingredients:

2 tablespoons olive oil

2 pounds ground chicken

1 red bell pepper, diced

1 green bell pepper, diced

1 onion, diced

1 (8-ounce) can diced water chestnuts, drained

2 cups cooked rice

3/4 cup teriyaki sauce, homemade or store-bought

2 heads butter lettuce

2 green onions, thinly sliced

1 teaspoon sesame seeds

Instructions

1. Heat olive oil in a saucepan over medium high heat. Add ground chicken and cook until browned, about 3-5 mins, making sure to crumble the chicken as it cooks; drain excess fat.

2. Place ground chicken, bell peppers, onion, water chestnuts and rice into a 6-qt slow cooker. Stir in teriyaki sauce.
3. Cover and cook on low heat for 3-4 hours or high heat for 1-2 hours.
4. To serve, spoon several tablespoons of the chicken mixture into the center of a lettuce leaf, taco-style, garnished with green onions and sesame seeds, if desired.

Vegetarian "Bone" Broth

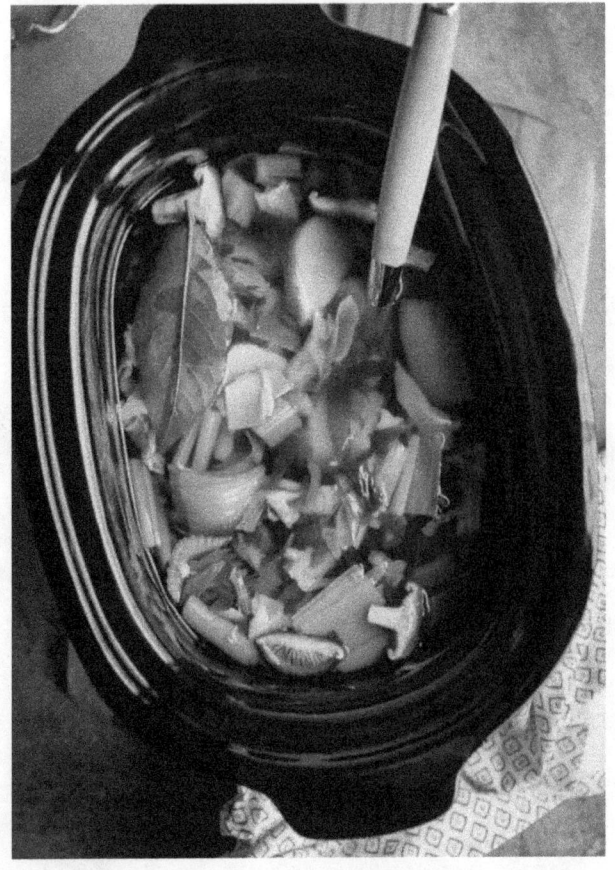

Full of minerals, vitamins, and other nutrients, this vegetarian "bone" broth is easy to make and can be consumed as-is or used as the base for soups and stews, and more to add extra nutrition and flavor.

Prep Time: 20 mins

Cook Time: 8 hrs

Total Time: 16 hrs 20 mins

Ingredients

2 cups fresh leafy greens cabbage, kale, collards, etc., chopped (stems too, if desired)

1 bunch carrots with tops if desired

4 celery stalks roughly chopped

1 medium sweet potato scrubbed well and cut into thick slices

1 large fennel bulb halved

1-2 medium onions halved

1 large leek root end trimmed, halved lengthwise and rinsed well

6-8 fresh shiitake mushrooms sliced (or a small package dried)

2 inches fresh ginger peeled and cut into thick slices

2 inches fresh turmeric peeled and cut into thick slices (or 2 teaspoons ground turmeric)

5-6 garlic cloves

2 bay leaves

3 tablespoons wakame

3 tablespoons coconut aminos

Herbs and spices optional

12-16 cups filtered water

Instructions

1. Wash and rinse all veggies well before slicing or chopping. Place in a large stockpot or slow cooker. Add the ginger, turmeric, garlic cloves, bay leaves, wakame, coconut aminos, and any other herbs or spices. Cover with the water.

2. If using the stove and a stockpot, bring to a boil, then lower heat to a simmer. Cover pot and cook for 2-3 hours. If using a slow cooker, cover with lid and turn on to HIGH for 6-8 hours or overnight. (Note: I don't like using LOW heat when using my slow cooker for broth. It should be simmering and I've only had that happen when I've used HIGH heat.)

3. With a slotted spoon, remove the solids from the pot or slow cooker. Set a large fine mesh strainer over a big bowl or another pot and strain the broth. If not using immediately, transfer the broth to jars or other airtight containers. Let cool slightly before placing in fridge or freezer. Broth should keep well for about 3-5 days in the fridge and several months in the freezer.

4. This broth has very little salt (except for the aminos), so add salt to taste according to how it will be used in recipes.

Notes

- Feel free to substitute or add any vegetables you have on hand or prefer over the ones listed above.
- Variation: for a tomato-based broth, add in 2-3 large tomatoes, halved or chopped
- Add in various spices and herbs according to how it will be used in recipes or according to preference. Example: thyme, parsley, sage, and rosemary for savory recipes; or cilantro, cumin seeds, and chili peppers for Mexican or Indian recipes, etc.

Pork Ramen

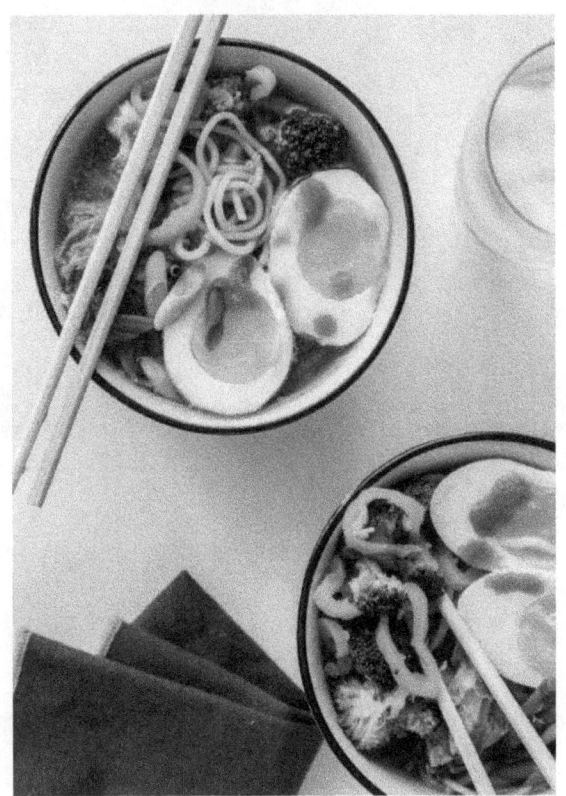

Yield: 8-10 servings

Prep Time: 15 mins

Cook Time: 8 hours

Total Time: 8 hours 15 mins

Ingredients

For The Broth

2 tablespoons vegetable oil

2-3 lb pork shoulder

salt and pepper

6 cups low sodium chicken broth (or vegetable or pork)

2 cups water

2 inch piece of ginger, peeled and sliced

1 onion, roughly chopped

1 stalk celery, cut in half

1 carrot, peeled and cut in quarters

1/4 cup white miso

1/4 cup low sodium soy sauce

3 garlic cloves, peeled and cut in half

1 tablespoon peppercorns

For Serving

ramen noodles, cooked (can use instant but discard the seasoning package)

steamed broccoli (or other veggies)

soft boiled eggs

sliced green onions

sriracha

soy sauce

Directions

Make The Broth

Heat oil in a cast iron skillet over medium high heat. Sprinkle pork shoulder with salt and pepper. Sear pork in cast iron skillet for about 2-3 mins per side. Place pork in slow cooker. Add remaining broth ingredients. Cook on low for 7-8 hours until the pork is extremely tender and falling apart. Remove pork and shred. Strain broth to remove all the solids.

Build The Bowls

Prepare the toppings while the broth is cooking. To build a bowl, place noodles in the bottom of a bowl and ladle broth on top. Top each bowl with a shredded pork, broccoli, soft boiled eggs, sliced green onions and a splash of sriracha and soy sauce. Serve and enjoy!

Chicken

Honey Teriyaki Chicken

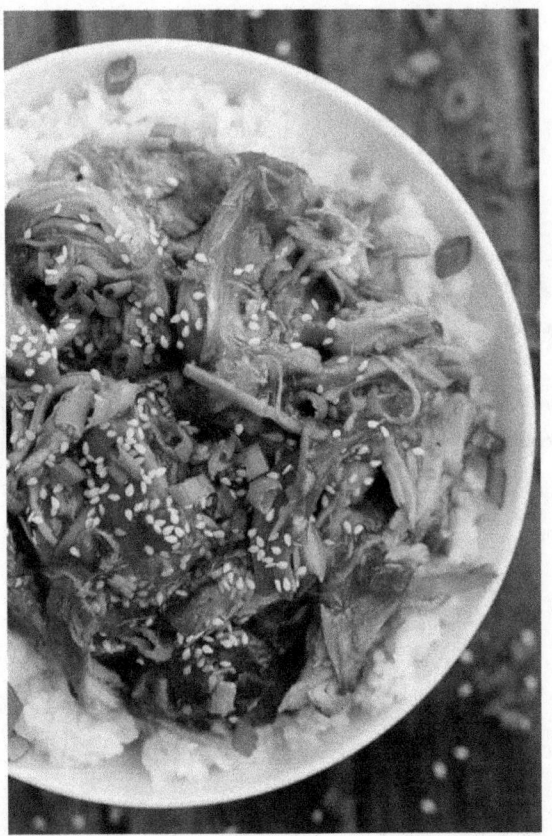

Prep Time: 10 MINS

Slow Cooker: 4 HOURS

Total Time: 4 HOURS 10 MINS

Servings: 6

This recipe is so easy to throw into your slow cooker and the honey teriyaki flavor is our of this world! The chicken cooks to perfection and will be one of the best things that you will make!

Ingredients

4 chicken breasts boneless, about 2 pounds

1/2 cup soy sauce

1/2 cup honey

1/4 cup rice wine vinegar

1/4 cup onion chopped

2 garlic cloves minced

1/4 teaspoon pepper

3/4 teaspoon ground ginger

1/4 cup water

3 Tablespoons Cornstarch

Optional garnish: green onions sesame seeds

Instructions

1. Spray your slow cooker with cooking spray and place the chicken breasts in the bottom. In a small bowl whisk the soy

sauce, honey, rice wine vinegar, onion, garlic, pepper and ginger. Pour over the chicken breasts.
2. Cook on high for 3-4 hours or low for 4-5 or until chicken is cooked throughout and shreds easily. Once the chicken is cooked, remove with a slotted spoon and shred on a plate.
3. Pour the sauce into a medium sauce pan. In a small bowl, whisk together the water and cornstarch. Slowly whisk into the sauce on medium high heat. Continue to whisk and let it boil until the honey teriyaki sauce starts to thicken. About 2 mins.
4. Add the chicken back to the slow cooker and pour the sauce on top stirring to coat. Serve over rice and garnish if desired.

Orange Chicken

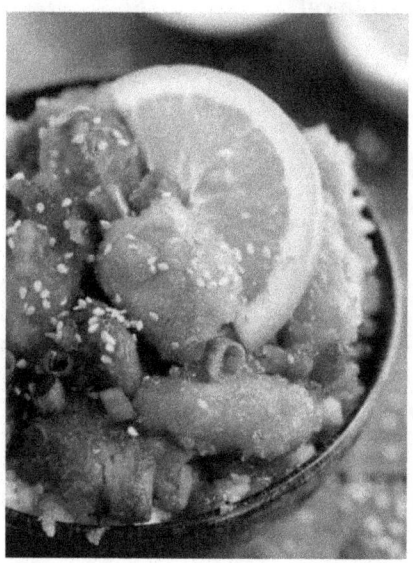

Prep Time: 15 MINS

Cook Time: 4 HOURS

Total Time: 4 HOURS 15 MINS

Servings: 4

A delicious and tangy orange chicken that is made right in your slow cooker! This is better than takeout and a meal that the entire family will love!

Ingredients

3-4 Boneless Chicken Breasts chopped into small pieces

3 Tablespoons Cornstarch

2 Tablespoons vegetable oil

1 teaspoon rice wine vinegar

2 Tablespoons Soy Sauce

1/2 teaspoon sesame oil

3/4 cup orange marmalade

3 Tablespoon brown sugar

1/2 teaspoon salt

pinch of pepper

Instructions

1. In a bowl mix the rice wine vinegar, soy sauce, sesame oil, marmalade, brown sugar, salt and pepper. Set aside.
2. In a ziplock bag, add the cornstarch and chicken. Shake to coat. Pour vegetable oil in the skillet and brown the sides of the covered chicken. The chicken doesn't need to be fully cooked since it is going in the crockpot.
3. After the chicken is done cooking, pour the pieces into the crockpot. Then cover the chicken with the sauce mixture and give the pot a stir.
4. Cook on low 4-5 hours or high 2-3 hours.

Cashew Chicken

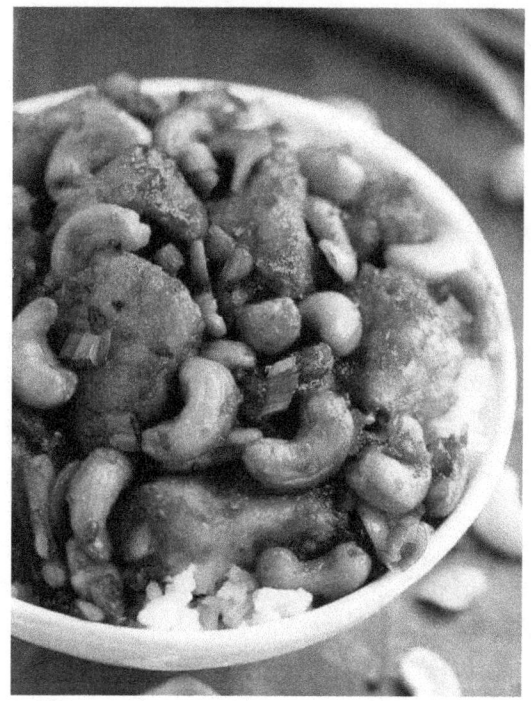

Prep Time: 15 MINS

Slow Cooker: 4 HOURS

Total Time: 4 HOURS 15 MINS

Servings: 6

An amazing slow cooker meal that is way better than takeout! The chicken is breaded to perfection and the sauce is full of flavor! The cashews hidden throughout are the best part!

Ingredients

2 lbs chicken breasts boneless skinless, About 4 pieces, cut into 1 inch pieces

3 Tablespoons Cornstarch

1/2 tsp black pepper

1 Tbsp canola oil

1/2 cup soy sauce low sodium

4 Tbsp rice wine vinegar

4 Tablespoons ketchup

2 Tablespoons sweet chili sauce

2 Tbsp brown sugar

2 garlic cloves minced

1 tsp grated fresh ginger

1/4 tsp red pepper flakes

1 cup cashews

Instructions

1. Combine cornstarch and pepper in resealable food storage bag.

Add chicken. Shake to coat with cornstarch mixture.

2. Heat oil in skillet over medium-high heat. Brown chicken about 2 mins on each side. Place chicken in slow cooker.
3. Combine soy sauce, vinegar, ketchup, sweet chili sauce sugar, garlic, ginger, pepper flakes, and cashews in small bowl; pour over chicken. (I like my cashews to be softer so I add them during the cooking process, if you want more of a crunch, add them right before serving)
4. Cook on LOW for 3 to 4 hours.
5. Serve over rice. Makes 4-6 servings.

Hainanese Chicken

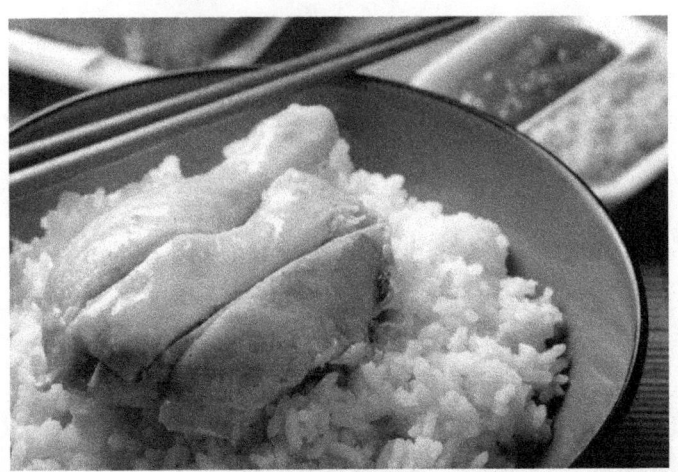

Prep Time: 15 mins

Cook Time: 5 hours

Total Time: 10 hours 15 mins

Ingredients

1 Whole Chicken

1 Bunch Pandan Leaves

1 Thumb-sized Ginger peeled, sliced

1 Bulbs garlic peeled, crushed

Salt

Chili Sauce optional

For the Ginger Dipping Sauce

1/4 Cup Ginger peeled, sliced

1 Bulb garlic peeled, crushed

1/4 Cup Sesame Oil

2 Tablespoons Poaching Stock

Instructions

1. Blanch chicken for about a minute in salted boiling water.
2. Rinse chicken under cold running water.
3. Combine chicken, pandan leaves, garlic, ginger, salt, and water in slow cooker. Cook for 4-6 hours on low.
4. Prepare ginger dipping sauce. Process ginger, garlic, sesame oil, stock, and salt in a food processor.

Meat

Slow Cooker Broccoli Beef

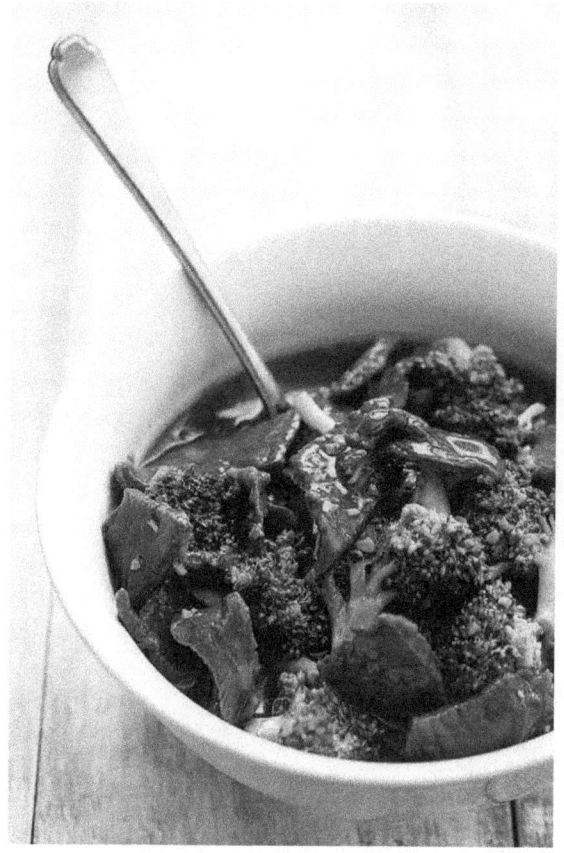

Prep Time: 10 MINS

Cook Time: 4 HOURS

Total Time: 4 HOURS 10 MINS

Servings: 4

Ingredients

1 1/2 pounds flank steak, thinly sliced and chopped into 2 inch pieces

1 cup beef broth

2/3 cup low sodium soy sauce

1/3 cup brown sugar

1 tablespoon sesame oil

1 tablespoon minced garlic

1/4 teaspoon red chili flakes (optional)

4 cups broccoli florets

2 tablespoons cornstarch

4 tablespoons cold water

Instructions

1. Grease the inside of a slow cooker. Add steak, beef broth, soy sauce, brown sugar, sesame oil, garlic, and chili flakes. Cover and cook on high for 2-3 hours or low 4-5 hours.
2. Mins before serving, uncover the slow cooker. In a small bowl, whisk corn starch and water until dissolved. Add to slow

cooker and stir. Cover and allow to cook another 20-25 mins.

3. Just before serving, place broccoli in a large tupperware, fill with 1/2 inch of water, and place the lid on in an off-set manner so that the container can vent. Microwave on high for 3 mins. Drain, stir broccoli into slow cooker, and serve.

Notes

- For a bit of a spicy kick, add a full 1-2 teaspoons of crushed red pepper flakes

Soy-Miso Glazed Beef Short Ribs

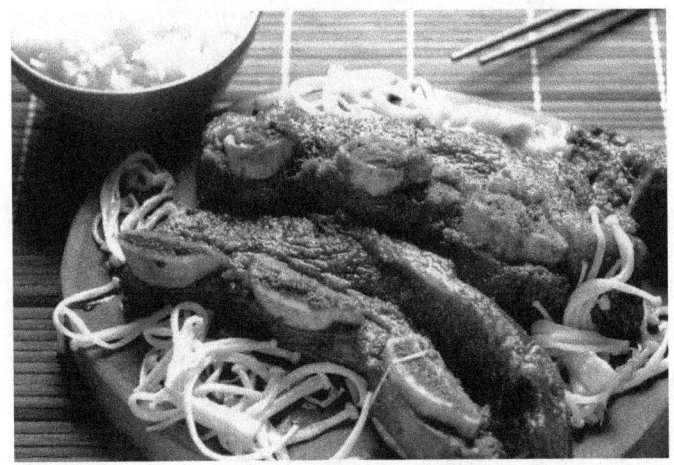

Prep Time: 15 mins

Cook Time: 8 hours

Total Time: 16 hours 15 mins

Ingredients

1.5 Kilograms Beef Short Ribs

1/2 Cup Soy Sauce

1/2 Cup Miso Paste

1/4 Cup Honey

1/4 Cup Rice Wine Vinegar

1 1/2 Cups Beef Stock

1 Pieces White Onion peeled, diced

1 Piece Carrot peeled, diced

1 Tablespoon Ginger grated

1 Bulb garlic finely chopped

1 Tablespoon Black Peppercorns crushed

Instructions

1. Combine soy sauce, miso paste, honey, ginger, garlic, rice wine vinegar, and black pepper into a paste.
2. Rub this paste to the beef ribs and marinate overnight.
3. Season beef with salt.
4. Sear the beef ribs in a pan then set aside.
5. Add the carrots and onions and roast briefly.
6. Deglaze pan with some stock.
7. Transfer all contents of the pan to the slow cooker.
8. Add beef and beef stock.
9. Cook on low for 8 hours.
10. Set aside beef ribs and reduce braising liquid to make the glaze.
11. Brush beef with the reduced glaze before serving.

Slow Cooker Sesame Beef

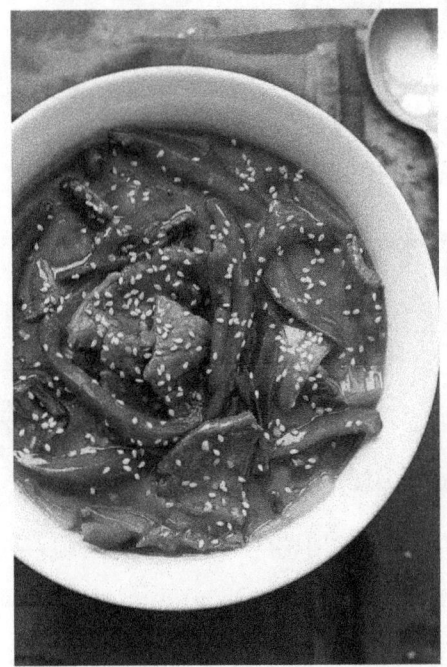

Prep Time: 10 MINS

Cook Time: 4 HOURS

Total Time: 4 HOURS 10 MINS

Servings: 4

Ingredients

16 ounces thin flank steak*, chopped into 2-inch pieces

1/2 white onion, chopped

1/4 cup sliced green onions

Sauce

3 tablespoons sesame oil

1 tablespoon minced garlic

1 red pepper, seeded and thinly sliced

3 tablespoons soy sauce

2 tablespoons brown sugar

1 tablespoon rice vinegar

1/2 cup water

1/2 teaspoon crushed red pepper

1/4 cup cold water

1 tablespoon corn starch

sesame seeds for garnish

Get IngredientsPowered by Chicory

Instructions

1. Place beef, onions (green and white), and chopped red peppers in a greased slow cooker.

2. In a medium bowl whisk together all sauce ingredients (do not include the 1/4 cup cold water, corn starch, or sesame seeds). Pour sauce into the slow cooker and stir to combine. Cover and cook 2-3 hours on high or 4-5 hours on low.
3. About 30 mins before serving, whisk together remaining cold water and corn starch. Add corn starch slurry to the slow cooker and stir. Cover and cook on high for another 30 mins or so. Stir just before serving. Serve with cooked white or fried rice and sprinkle with sesame seeds.

Notes

- The thinner the beef you use, the more tender it will be after it's finished cooking. Try to look for flank steak or similar beef product that has been sliced very thin.*For serving, click [url:1]here[/url] for my favorite fried rice recipe and [url:2]here[/url] for super easy chicken fried rice!

Slow Cooker Sweet & Sour Meatballs

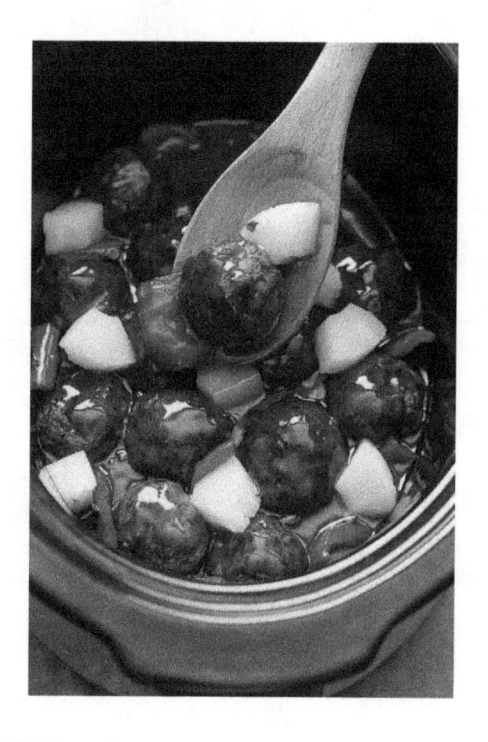

Prep Time: 15 MINS

Cook Time: 3 HOURS

Total Time: 3 HOURS 15 MINS

Servings: 4

Saucy sweet and sour meatballs with red peppers and pineapple made right in your crockpot!

Ingredients

1-2 pounds lean ground beef (non-lean works too)

1 egg + 1 egg yolk

1/2 cup bread crumbs

1 teaspoon salt

1/2 teaspoon pepper

2 teaspoons garlic powder

2 teaspoons onion powder

1 cup pineapple chunks, drained (not crushed)

1 red pepper, seeded, stem removed, and chopped

Sauce

3/4 cup sugar

1/2 cup apple cider vinegar (may sub white vinegar)

2 tablespoons soy sauce

1 teaspoon garlic powder

1/2 teaspoon onion powder

1/4 cup ketchup

1/2 teaspoon crushed red pepper flakes (optional)

1 tablespoon cornstarch

2 tablespoons cold water

Instructions

1. In a large bowl combine ground beef, egg and yolk, breadcrumbs, salt, pepper, garlic powder, and onion powder. Use your hands to mash everything together until the ingredients are well-mixed. Roll the mixture into 1.5 inch balls. Place meatballs side by side in a single layer in the bottom of a greased crockpot. Add pineapple chunks (without juice) and red peppers.
2. Prepare the sauce by whisking together sugar, apple cider vinegar, soy sauce, garlic powder, onion powder, ketchup, and red pepper flakes in a bowl. Pour over meatballs in the crockpot. Cover and cook on high for 1-2 hours or on low 3-4 hours.
3. About 30 mins before serving, in a small bowl whisk together cold water and corn starch. Pour into crockpot and stir. Cover and allow to thicken for about 30 mins before serving. Sprinkle with sesame seeds if desired.

Notes

- Alternate oven cooking method: instead of placing meatballs in the slow cooker, place them on a greased baking sheet along with the chopped red peppers. Bake them for 15-20 mins until cooked though and browned. Remove from oven and add to a large sauce pan with your sweet and sour sauce, the cooked red peppers, and the pineapple chunks and stir over medium heat. Add the corn starch slurry and allow to thicken for about 5 mins before serving.

Slow Cooker Asian Pulled Pork

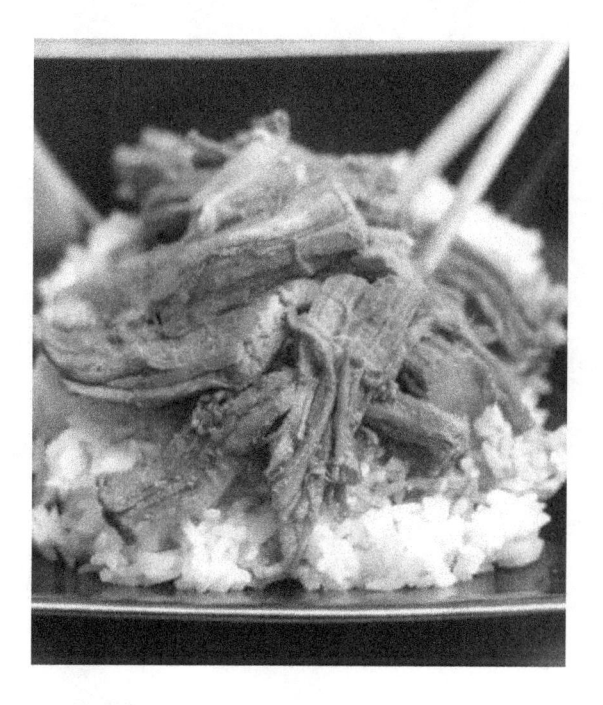

Prep Time: 15 MINS

Cook Time: 8 HOURS

Total Time: 8 HOURS 15 MINS

Servings: 6

Ingredients

2-3 pounds of pork roast

1 cup water

1/2 tsp Shirley J Chicken bouillon or 1 tsp chicken bouillon granules

1 onion cut into large chunky slices

1/4 cup low sodium soy sauce

1 Tbsp Worcestershire Sauce

1 tsp minced garlic

1 Tbsp brown sugar

2 Tbsp Oyster Sauce

Instructions

1. Spray slow cooker with cooking spray and place the pork on the bottom. Pour the water and bouillon. Place onions around the roast. Cover and cook on low 7-10 hours. The pork should be tender and easy to shred.
2. When pork is finished drain the juices and discard onions. Shred the meat.
3. Combine soy sauce, Worchestershire, garllic, brown sugar and oyster sauce. Pour over the meat and stir.
4. Let it cook for another 30 mins so that the flavors are blended.
5. Serve over hot rice or ramen noodles.

Vegetables & Tofu

Slow Cooked Asian Vegetables

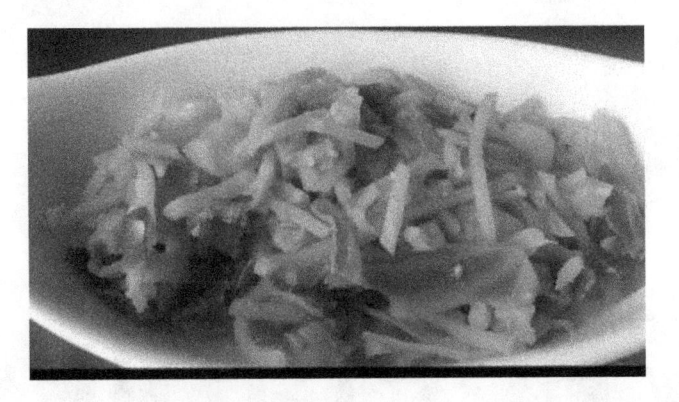

Quick and easy vegetable side dish

Prep: 10 mins

Cook: 30 mins

Yields: 8 as a side dish

Ingredients

800g of shredded stir-fry vegetables (you can buy them packaged in produce section or shred your own)

- Red Cabbage

- White Cabbage

- Wombok

- Carrot

- Broccoli

- Spring Onion/Shallots

1 cup salt reduced liquid vegetable stock

1 heaped teaspoon minced garlic

1 heaped teaspoon minced ginger

1-2 tablespoons of Maggi Original Seasoning (It's an Asian flavour similar to soy sauce)

Directions

1. Combine all ingredients in slow cooker
2. Cook the first 10mins on searing/HIGH
3. Stir through to combine the liquid and vegetables again
4. Then turn it down to slow cook on LOW for an additional 20mins

Notes

- Served as a side dish to BBQ steak and it was delicious and easy
- Vegetable volume could be halved to serve 4 if desired

Slow Cooker Asian Greens (gluten free)

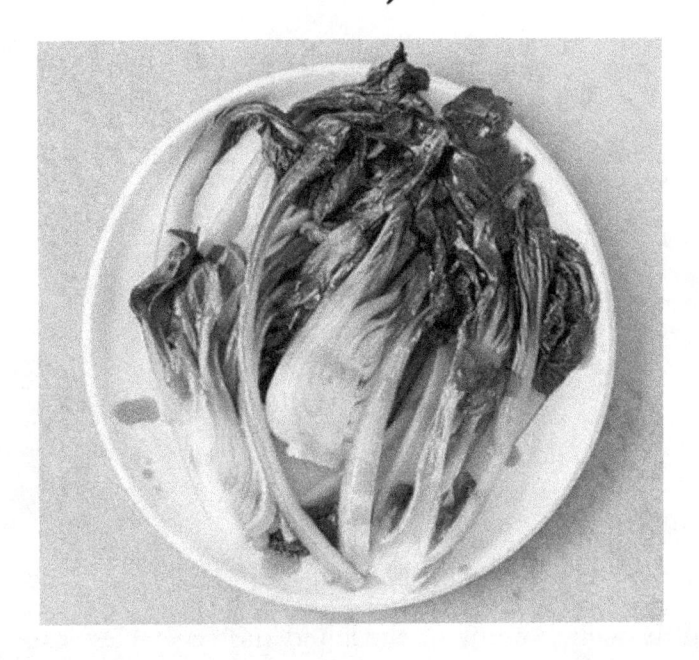

Use a 1 – 2 quart slow cooker for this one – (or multiply recipe and use larger one)

Prep Time: 10 mins

Cook Time: 7 hrs

Total Time: 7 hrs 10 mins

Ingredients

1 bunch greens of your choice or mix and match: collards, kale,

turnip greens, beet greens, etc.

1 clove garlic minced

1 tsp ginger grated

1 Tb soy sauce * gluten free people make sure you have gluten-free soy sauce or add some salt instead

1 tsp rice wine vinegar you can substitute white vinegar if you don't have any

1/4 to 1/2 cup water if cooking all day

sesame oil or chili sesame oil to taste

Instructions

The night before:

1. Wash and cut up the greens.
2. Mince the garlic and grate the ginger.

In the morning:

1. Put everything except the sesame oil in the slow cooker and cook on low for 8 hours. (Or on high for 4 hours.)
2. Top with sesame oil. Use chili oil for more of a kick.

Orange-Teriyaki Tofu

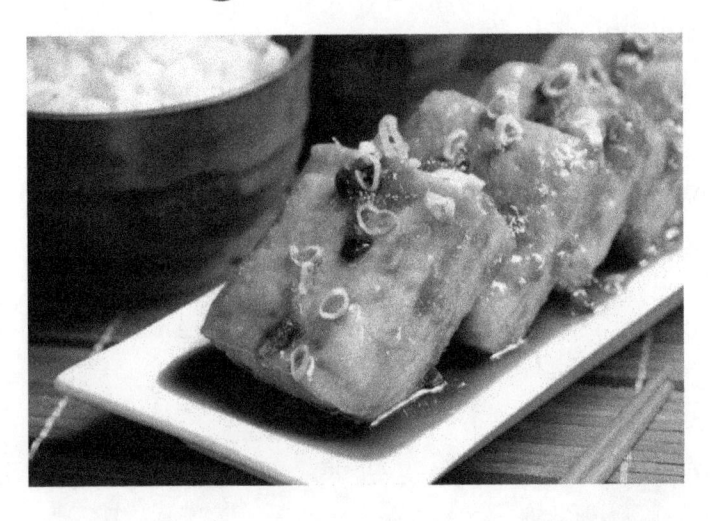

This simple tofu dish is proof that vegan dishes can definitely be tasty. Well, that's how it should be – going on a plant-based diet shouldn't come with giving up on the pleasure of eating as well.

Prep Time: 10 mins

Cook Time: 4 hours

Total Time: 8 hours 10 mins

Ingredients

500 Grams Firm Tofu

1 Tablespoon Grated Ginger

1/4 Cup Fresh Orange Juice

1/4 Cup Sugar

1/4 Cup Soy Sauce

1 Bunch Leeks thinly sliced

Instructions

1. Combine ginger, orange juice, sugar, soy sauce, and leeks in a bowl.
2. Pan fry tofu on both sides.
3. Combine tofu and sauce in the slow cooker and leave on a low setting for 4 hours.

Tofu Lo Mein

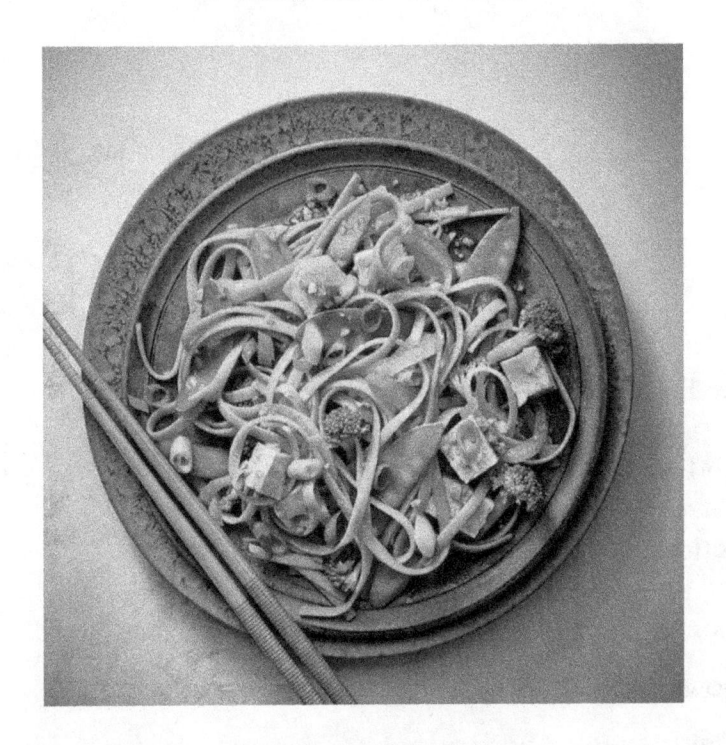

Crisp-tender veggies cooked in a sweet Asian sauce and served with noodles and tofu is a refreshingly different slow cooker dinner. Removing the excess moisture from the tofu helps it soak up the sauce, giving the unassuming ingredient full flavor.

Active: 30 mins

Total: 2 hrs 30 mins

Servings: 5

Ingredients

Ingredient Checklist

1 yellow onion (about 8 ounces), thinly sliced

2 cups fresh broccoli florets (from 1 head broccoli)

1 cup diagonally sliced carrots (about 4 1/2 ounces)

1 (8 ounce) package fresh snow peas, trimmed

⅔ cup unsalted vegetable stock

¼ cup sliced scallions (from 2 scallions)

3 tablespoons lower-sodium soy sauce

3 tablespoons oyster sauce

2 tablespoons rice vinegar

1 tablespoon minced fresh ginger

1 tablespoon sesame oil

2 teaspoons honey

3 garlic cloves, minced (about 1 tablespoon)

8 ounces uncooked whole-wheat linguine

1 (14 ounce) package extra-firm tofu, drained

Instructions

1. Place the onions, broccoli, carrots, and snow peas in a 4- to 5-quart slow cooker. Whisk together the stock, scallions, soy sauce, oyster sauce, vinegar, ginger, oil, honey, and garlic; pour over the vegetables in the slow cooker. Cover and cook on LOW until the vegetables are tender, 2 to 3 hours.
2. Meanwhile, cook the pasta to al dente according to the package directions. Drain well.
3. Place the tofu on several layers of paper towels; cover with additional paper towels. Press to absorb the excess moisture; cut into 1/2-inch cubes.
4. Add the tofu and the hot cooked linguine to the slow cooker, stirring to combine.